Table of Contents

Dedication

This collection is dedicated to the wonderful parents on the Pediatric and Adolescent Migraine and Headache Disorders Parent Support Group on Facebook, who have been a lifeline to me. They truly understand the victory it can be when a kid can make it to the shower.
It is a thank you to the outstanding caregivers at the Cleveland Clinic who have worked with my son.
It is to my amazing, resilient son who I admire more than I can say. And it is with deepest love to my husband, who takes my son from our door to the school's every morning I can help him move from bed to doorway.

Preface
June 27, 2016

I am a developmental psychologist who studies parent-adolescent relationships for a living. That's not where this is coming from. This is from me as a mom. A mom who has spent much of the last several years struggling with pain. Not my pain, but my son's. That makes it worse.

My son has severe chronic migraines. It started out of the blue. In sixth grade, after an almost illness-free childhood, he suddenly felt a little sick. No big deal – it seemed like a stomach bug. But that stomach bug turned into frequent nausea and rounds of tests that confirmed nothing. Then they said it was 'anxiety' because nothing was 'wrong' but he was vomiting constantly. Then the migraines started. First a few days a month. Then a few days a week. Then weeks and weeks and weeks of pain, where the sound of a cat walking across the floor would cause him to dive, whimpering, under the covers, where the flicker of an iPod would cause him to wince, and where my first thought every morning was 'how bad is it going to be today?'.

Different people cope differently with the agony of having a child in pain. I look for information and, because I was already a blogger for **Psychology Today** I also write.

This is a collection of some of the pieces I've written while taking this journey. I am not an expert in pain. I'm just a mom.

Section I
Kids Who Go To School In Pain

Children Who Go To School In Pain

Thousands of children go to school in pain every day[a]

Let me tell you about my morning

I guess my morning started last night. Maybe it started a few months ago.

For the last several months, my son, like clockwork, gets a migraine on Sunday afternoon. It starts with him feeling a little odd and spacey. Then he would start getting flashing lights in front of his eyes. Sometimes the whole room he is looking at distorts, like one of those weird spatial anomalies in Star Trek.

Then the pain starts. Sharp stabbing pain through the top his head (ice pick headaches), the thudding at the base of his neck, and the pressure at both temples.

But the worse part are the sensitivities. Wincing from the unbearable noise of the cat walking across the room or the birds singing outside or the radio on three rooms away. And cringing from the light in the hallway. Did you know you can feel pain when someone just puts their hand 3" over the top of your skull? You can. It feels like deep, unrelenting pressure.

And the nausea. And vertigo.

Last spring, the migraine would start Sunday and leave Thursday or Friday. In June, there were three days when he didn't have a migraine. After months of special diets and medications, we're down to Sundays. Every Sunday starting between 2:30 and 4:00. And it's actually been getting much better – usually ending by bedtime or by morning. We had been feeling a glimmer of hope.

So yesterday, we were really happy when he got all the way until 6:00 before it started. Unfortunately, this morning it was still there. The pain was a little less, but with full bore vomiting until there was nothing left and he had the dry heaves. Thankfully, no sensitivities.

After feeding him a breakfast he immediately lost, I packed him up, helped him get dressed, and pushed him out the door to school. It is the hardest thing I have ever had to do - as a parent or otherwise - packing him out the door when he's so obviously in pain. But his neurologist and the pain specialist say it's like physical therapy and will help retrain his brain. His brain needs to learn that light and sound and breezes on his face aren't pain. And they're right: school helps him. And my son knows they're right. But he still doesn't want to go. And I don't blame him.

Children in School with Chronic Pain

In the last few months, I've met a lot of parents with kids who are in pain like this. Or much worse pain.

> Through a friend, I met a woman whose 16 year old was hit on the head with softball and has been in unbearable pain - like the worst of my son's migraines - for over four years. She just started college this fall.

> I've looked at adorable pictures of a toddler running around with sound cancelling headphones because when she gets migraines, she cries uncontrollably from the normal sounds of a household. With the headphones on she can run around her bedroom.

> I've listened to parents talking about bringing their kids in for 33 botox shots every 3 months to reduce chronic daily headaches from 20 days a month to only a few days a week. Others trying nerve decompression surgery to stop pain in pre-adolescents that has gone on for two or four or five years. Experimental surgery and medicines on top of the chiropractic sessions, massage, herbal remedies, diet changes, meditation, and exercise which all help some people.

Some of these kids have congenital problems. Some have suffered concussions or been in car crashes. All of them are in pain, many of them for years on end.

Reconciling Pain With School

Just like parents with children with cognitive or physical disabilities have things they just get tired of people saying, there are things that parents with children with headaches get tired of hearing.

- I've had a few migraines too. I can sympathize. (A two hour migraine - no matter how bad - doesn't help you fully understand what it's like to have that kind of pain day after day, week after week, sometimes for years at a time. It just doesn't.)
- Can't they just work through the pain? (No. If they could, they would)
- Are you sure they're not faking it? (Yes.)
- Have you tried Excedrin Migraine/Alleve/Tylenol . . . ? (Yes. Do you know that many chronic headaches are caused by overuse of over-the-counter medications that are designed to be taken rarely, but not for ongoing pain?)

And my least favorite: Maybe you're just putting too much pressure on them. A lot of kids get headaches from stress. Just what I need: to be told it's all my fault. It's bad enough I can't fix it when all I want is to take the pain from him. It would be so much easier to carry it myself. Chronic headaches and migraines are not caused by stress. These types of headaches are caused by a neurological problem or problems. Stress can make them worse - just like stress makes it more likely you will become ill with a virus. But stress is not the cause. Experiencing headaches and pain is very stressful, however.

Catch-22: Faking Being Well

The kids also get in this Catch-22.

If they go to school in pain, they often get really good at hiding it. They laugh and joke. They walk around. They talk to friends. They don't usually cry. They vomit secretly in the bathroom so that they won't get sent home. They try to participate in extracurricular activities to distract themselves from pain. And the more normal they look, the more likely it is that people will see them acting normally and decide they're just faking it.

Dealing With Chronic Illness Isn't The Same As Dealing With a Short Term Illness

We are blessed with a school nurse who really does understand what serious, chronic migraines are like. We have an understanding school district and my son has very many patient, concerned teachers. But let me tell you one more reason why being chronically ill is different than being out with the flu for two weeks or having a broken leg or having mono.

It never goes away. Think of what that means for schoolwork, which also never goes away. It means when my son goes to school in pain, he works slowly and suffers from difficulties focusing. He is absent minded and disorganized, like people are after a concussion or a seizure. His brain isn't working right. That's why he has a migraine. So his school work doesn't get done.

He comes home from a day at school in pain, with all his regular homework and all the extra work from school he didn't complete.

He spends his weekends making up the work from the week before.

When his migraines really get going, he is always in pain or making up the work he couldn't do when he was in pain. He never gets a day off. He never gets to relax. He never gets to just kick back and do nothing. Or when he does, he knows it's going to cost him. Because there's always more work he should be doing. And then he worries about that. Which makes him stressed. Which can, in fact, trigger migraines. Or he can't sleep. Which can, in fact, trigger migraines.

With incredibly willpower he has not missed a day of school after the first week because of migraines. He's gone to school in pain. He's gone to school vomiting. He has gone to school when he was whimpering from the sound of the pigeons outside his bedroom window.

And when he got the flu, he missed two weeks of school. And now he has more work to make up.

There are tens of thousands of kids in this country who suffer from migraines. There are others with concussions that cause chronic pain. There are kids with congenital spine defects that stop the normal flow of spinal fluid and cause excruciating pain. There are kids with chiari malformation. There are lots of kids in pain for lots of different reasons. There are parents all over the world who are coping with this and children with many other forms of invisible, chronic diseases.

They deserve admiration, support, and as creative solutions for their problems as we can find.

Getting Kids in Pain to School: Tips From the Trenches

School helps kids in pain. But how do you get them there?[a]

My youngest son lives with severe, frequent pain. He has chronic migraines. In the last 35 days, he's been pain free for five of them. This morning he would squeal with the sound of a toilet flushing in another room, shudder when the light hit his face, and lie shaking at the prospect of just sitting up in bed.

Think of an ice cream headache that lasts for four days. Then starts again.

I have written before about children who to go school in pain. Chronic pain is counter-intuitive. First of all, it seems impossible that anyone could live in that much pain all the time. Second, it seems implausible that people who are in a lot of pain can look normal, act as if they're okay, or laugh and talk with friends. They can, it just takes a lot of practice and uses a lot of energy.

Neuropathic pain is dysfunctional in that the pain itself is the disease. The nerves start firing and don't stop. Curing the disease requires quieting and retraining the nerves. The most recommended way to do that is to return to functioning. That means getting up and living your life. This does not mean 'pushing through' your pain. I hate that phrase. It implies that if you just try hard enough, the pain will go away. It doesn't - at least not short term. I prefer to think about it the way they talk about it at the Cleveland Clinic Pediatric Pain Rehab program:

You are in a lot of pain. That pain isn't going away right now. You can curl up on the couch and embrace it. Or you can take it with you and try to live your life.

Why Should Kids In Pain Go To School?

For kids, that means going to school in pain. Research suggests that compared to kids who withdraw and are home schooled, kids who go back to school despite chronic pain reduce the number of days they experience pain and reduce their experienced pain. They also become less chronically ill from other diseases. Lying in bed for weeks, months, and years because it hurts too much to get up makes you physically weak. And weak bodies are prone to disease. It makes you depressed. And depression reduces your immune system's ability to keep you well. And it means the child is not doing the other important tasks that kids need to do: play, learn, and be with others.

PLEASE NOTE: If your child is anxious as well as in pain, you are facing a much more difficult situation and want to work even more closely with a therapist who is skilled in dealing with these issues. The techniques described here and the links below will be helpful, but may have to be modified for your special circumstances. All kids are different. That said . . .
.

People in pain need help. I think of functioning with pain as physical therapy for the brain. And physical therapy is often painful. As I have written before, if your child has this type of pain, they need help dealing with it. Stress reduction techniques, breathing techniques, and biofeedback can help reduce the experience of pain and help you to cope with it. A good pain therapist will also help you develop a concrete set of plans to put in place to deal with upcoming pain, coping with active pain, and dealing with the aftermath of your limited functionality during pain. And they can help with the frequent handmaidens of pain: depression and anxiety.

How To Get Them Out The Door?

When his doctors first told my son had to go to school in pain, I (1) didn't believe they could possibly be serious and (2) had no idea how to do it. They were. I now have too much experience.

One of the things I have learned through this experience is that it is very helpful to talk to other people who are going through the same thing. They provide support. They also know, collectively, a lot. Find a group. There are many on Facebook. There are more of us around than you think.

Tips for your child:

Set an expectation that they are going. You don't want to start every morning with an evaluation of whether they are bad enough to stay home.

They are not contagious. Staying home will not help them heal. Having an argument makes everyone more tense and tension makes pain worse. You both need to agree to this plan and commit to it.

Everyone has to be on board. Sending a kid in pain to school is incredibly wrenching. It goes against every one of my protective mom instincts. I can't tell you how many times I have done this with tears running down my face. You need the support of all family members. I am truly blessed in that my husband and I work together on this. I get my son to the door. He drives him to school and gets him in the door. Many people aren't that lucky. If you have a partner and they are undermining efforts to help your child function and heal—or worse, if they say the disease isn't real—this may be a time when family counseling is appropriate. At the minimum, they need to agree to get out of the way.

The foot in the door technique.

I wrote a full essay about this technique. The 'foot in the door' is a well established social psychology principle that if you say 'yes' to one thing, you are more likely to say 'yes' to the next request. So I don't start off a bad morning saying, 'get ready for school'. Some days that's too much. Instead, I start off saying 'can you sit up?' Then I ask him to go to the bathroom. Then put on shirt and pants. Then finally, we're going to the car. One step at a time, he gets into the car and into the school.

This is a technique he uses on himself, by the way, to get through the day once he's at school. At 10AM in overwhelming pain, the idea of staying to 3:30 seems impossible. But getting to lunch to see his friends? Making it to study hall so he can rest? Just getting through Spanish? And by then there's only an hour left so he might as well finish. And then there's a fun extracurricular —and if he forced himself to stay to work, he might as well stay for fun. One step at a time can take you a thousand miles.

The door in the face technique.

This is the opposite technique. You make a huge request—get dressed and get out the door. They balk. Back off. Can you get dressed? They may say yes.

Start early. Pain hurts and they need time to gird their loins, get their defenses up, and get ready to jump into the fray. An earlier wakeup time helps. Don't rush. Things are stressful enough already.

Remind them to use their skills. Hopefully, they have skills they can use to cope with pain. They are similar to ones used in childbirth education classes.

- BREATHE. Slow regular cleansing breaths help.
- VISUALIZATION. Imagine yourself on a beach listening to waves. Every wave washes across you gently, leaving you a little more relaxed.
- COUNTING. Focusing your mind on anything but the pain helps. Count tiles on the floor. How many red things are there in the room? What is 5 x 7? Using your brain gives it something to do that isn't suffering.
- RELAXATION. Consciously relax each muscle from the feet to the jaws and top of the head. Pain makes you tense. Tension increases pain. Consciously overcome it.
- SELF HYPNOSIS. Using self-hypnosis or biofeedback techniques are invaluable for removing yourself from the pain and relaxing. If you don't know how, find a clinician or practitioner to teach you.

Mindfulness. The only good thing about being hypersensitized to sensation is that it can make good sensations better too. Help them focus all their attention on that delicious orange they're biting into or the softness of their fleece jacket.
Hold them. They are never too old to be held. When I hug my very tense son I can feel his muscles relaxing. That's what he needs.

Ready, then relax. One of my newer insights is to change the order we do things in the morning. I used to have my son do his relaxation techniques. Then he'd get dressed, pack his backpack, then get out the door. On bad pain days, that made for a hectic morning and lost all the relaxation he needed to start his difficult day. Now, we get him fed and dressed first. Even shoes and (today) his coat. At that point he did his relaxation techniques. When it was time to hit the door, all he had to do was to come up from is 'trance' and walk to the car. Much less stress.

You need to breathe too

Helping a child do this is painful and difficult. You need to relax too. I do all those relaxation techniques with my child.

- **Talk softly, but firmly.** I always think of really good triage nurses. When your child is in pain, all they hear is your voice. It's their lifeline. Keep it steady.
- **Keep moving in a positive direction.**
- **It's okay to get frustrated**. But continue to recognize their pain and that it's not their fault. We're all frustrated with the pain. They're rather not do this either.
- **Use Rewards.** Kids Respond to Pleasure, Not Punishment.

The neuroscience of children and adolescent development is fascinating. One of the things that we've learned recently is that kids don't respond to threats—especially threats about negative consequences in the future. They're brains literally don't respond.

But boy do they respond to pleasure!

This can be helpful. In a post I did a few years ago, I talked about how this influenced my parenting.

Concretely, that means praising every single movement in the right direction, no matter how small. Each time they do something hard and are rewarded or acknowledged, it builds their sense of efficacy and their confidence that they can do more. Telling them that if they don't go to school they won't go to college is much less compelling than saying 'good' when they get up the energy to put their tee-shirt on.

No Easy Answers.

Some kids have complex problems and going to full day school is impossible for them. Some can make it for partial days. Some do homeschooling. But functioning is important.

Some days you try. Some days you make it. Some days you don't. But you keep moving forward.

Some days you run out of energy (spoons) and need to regroup.

But calm persistence and a bag of techniques can help them move in the right direction.

Getting Kids To Do Things: The Foot In The Door

Helping Kids To Do Things They'd Rather Not[1]

As I've written previously, my son frequently lives with severe pain. He has migraines, One of the many, many things that means for us as a family is that I spend a lot of time trying to get my son to do things he knows he has to do, but doesn't want to or just plain thinks he can't. These things aren't complicated. But when I say he doesn't want to, I mean getting him to do them is like getting a mule up a ladder backwards. The kid invented passive resistance. And he's a master of the active form.

The things he doesn't want to do can be mundane things like getting out of bed. Getting dressed. Taking a shower. Going to school.

They can be tedious but necessary things. Doing homework. Emptying the dishwasher. Feeding the chickens. Bringing in wood. The kinds of things no kid really wants to do even when they're feeling fine.

They can even be fun things. Going out for a hot dog. Walking on the beach. Watching a movie.

Nobody likes to fight with their kid, and fighting with a child who has a migraine is not only painful to you both, but counter-productive. So I've had to find other ways to help him do what he needs to do. Because part of my job as a parent is helping him get stuff done and continue to live his life.

A Foot In The Door

One of my most useful parenting tools is one familiar to anyone who has ever taken social psychology: the *Foot in the Door* technique.

The Foot in the Door technique is named after the sales technique used by door-to-door salesmen. They'd knock on your door and ask if you were interested in their brushes or vacuum cleaners. They'd ask a few simple questions. If they could get their foot in the door, odds were, they could make a sale.

The principle is simple. Every time someone asks you a question and you say 'yes', it increases the likelihood that you will say yes to the following question. One person who called me recently to give money to a charity was a master at this.

> Is this Nancy Darling?
> *Yes.*
> Hi, I'm calling from (well known charity). We provide services to people who have disabilities. Do you know anyone with a disability?
> *Yes*

You can imagine the rest of this conversation. They asked me about my acquaintance, asked if they used services, asked if they might be interested in the services provided by the charity . . . Then they asked if I might be willing to email my congressman to support their cause. Everything they said was designed to get me to answer a simple question - preferably with the answer 'yes'. And every time I did answer, it made it harder for me to refuse to answer, to say no, or to hang up. In other words, it increased the odds that when they finally asked me for money, I would say 'yes'.

In charity work, studies have shown that asking people to first express support (e.g., signing a petition) prior to asking for money markedly increases the likelihood that the person will make a donation (Schwarzwald, Bizman, and Raz, 1983). Interestingly, this is true even if the request for donation occurs two weeks after the petition was signed.

Why does this work? Researchers have argued that the primary reason is that saying 'yes' to the larger requests makes it easier for the person to remain internally consistent in their self-beliefs. So if I say I believe in a charity's work, it would be internally consistent with that belief to support them financially, and make me feel I was hypocritical if I said I supported them but did not donate money. In addition, each 'yes' helps to build a social connection between myself and the person making the request, although research suggests that this is less of a motivation than my own desire for internal consistency.

The Foot In The Door and Kids

This technique works for anyone - it is one of the most robust findings in the psychological literature. It even helps when persuading kids to do things they need to do but would rather not.

I used it this morning to help my son take a shower when he was in a huge amount of pain. He had been in bed under the covers, because the light was bothering his eyes and sound was painful. He wanted a shower, but it was too overwhelming. So we started small.

> Can you just sit up?
> *Yes* (He sat there for a minute.)
> Do you think you can stand?
> *Yes*
> How about just walking to the bathroom? (He made it that far.)
> I'm going to close the door. Do you think you can get undressed and take a shower?

Twenty minutes later he was showered. And feeling a little better.

He could not just get up and take a shower. But he could take little tiny steps, each of which was manageable. And even though the steps got bigger and bigger, every small step he had taken made it easier for him to tackle the next one. In fact, after his shower, he not only got dressed, but did get that hot dog and walk on a cold, wintry beach. Not bad for a kid who didn't know if he could sit up in bed.

The Door In the Face

What makes this an example of the Foot In The Door technique is that I started with small requests and each subsequent one got a little larger.

But if we stepped back another minute, this could be an example of another successful technique for gaining cooperation: the Door In The Face technique.

> Come have a hot dog with me and we'll go for a walk on the beach.
> *No, I can't.*
> Can you take a shower and get dressed?

The Door In the Face technique is simple. You ask someone to do something big (going for a hotdog and a walk) that you know they will refuse. When they say no to that, you make a much smaller request (taking a shower). Starting with a big request that is refused increases the likelihood that they say yes to the smaller one. Not as much as if you did the Foot In The Door, but more than just asking for the small request alone. Some research has found you et 100% compliance with Foot In The Door and around 80% for the smaller request in Door In The Face.

Increasing Effectiveness

The Foot in the Door works best when there is a little time between the first and second request. In other words, if I first said, "Can you sit up?" and then immediately said "Can you stand?" my second request would likely get a "no". A little time between requests helps, because it gives them time to think about what they've done and internalize it (I'm sitting up! I can do it!). Then when you make the new request, the belief that they can do things is more consistent with saying 'yes I can stand up' than with 'no I can't stand up'.

It Works For Homework Too

This afternoon - now that we've been out for that hot dog - he'll start his homework the same way. Starting with asking if he can find his books. Then finding his assignments. Then working for 5 minutes. Then finishing the first page. At some point I know he'll be lost in what he's doing and won't need all the little prompts.

But starting with very small commitments is an incredibly useful tool when the big ones just seem too overwhelming. It's an alternative to both yelling and to ineffective nagging by asking the same question over and over and over. And it might make both of you a little bit happier.

This piece wasn't written specifically for parenting a child in pain. But kids in pain often have trouble concentrating and the powerful drugs they take often make it even harder. If homework is a problem for your child, make sure their IEP or 504 addresses that issue specifically

Keep Your Middle Schooler Organized

Helping kids develop organizational skills relieves the homework struggle[·]

My youngest stomped into the living room last Monday and dumped his pack on the floor.

"How was school?"
"Great! I only have math homework."
I paused "Are you sure?"
"Absolutely. Nothing else. I asked my friend, too."
Didn't you have Spanish today?"
"Oh yeah, he gave us a worksheet to do. And we started our new technology class today. It looks great."
"Don't you usually have a syllabus or something to sign when you start a class?"
"Oh yeah, I forgot. I need you to sign two papers."
"It's Monday. Didn't you have a letter you had to write in class today in Language Arts? Do I need to sign it?"
"Yeah."
"And spelling due Thursday?"
"Uhuh. She handed out a sheet."
"Your social studies teacher sent me a copy of your study guide for your test Friday."
"But that's not due until Thursday!"

The Organizational Demands Of Middle School

Sound familiar? Five assignments. My son had only remembered one. And given that up to 75% of his grades are based on homework, not remembering to do it - or to turn it in when it's complete - can cause major problems for kids, failing grades, and even retention in middle school,

Middle school differs from elementary school in many ways - one of the most important, but underestimated, is the increased pressure it puts in kids' organizational abilities. Take the above example. Not only does it show off my son's not atypical difficulty keeping track of his work. It also shows up just how COMPLICATED the work is that he has to keep track of.

- Five courses with six different teachers
- Due dates of one, two, and four days.
- Different types of tasks, each needing different types of materials to complete them

Cognitive Development In Middle School

Although kids make major gains in cognitive ability as they enter adolescence, often the demands of school outstrip them. As I wrote in my previous post: What MIddle School Parents Should Know: Adolescents Are Like Lawyers, middle schoolers make five major gains in their ability to think:

- They can think about possibilities
- They can think about abstract concepts
- Their metacognitive abilities improve (they can think about thinking)
- They can think multi-dimensionally, playing one idea off of another
- They can think relativistically, understanding things from different points of views.
- The misfit on middle schools to early adolescents' development

A positive side of this development is that they are capable of much more abstract, multidimensional thinking.

Unfortunately, these new abilities often put them in conflict with the demands of middle schools.

Middle school requires more rote learning. As developmental researcher

Jacqueline Eccles has written, at the same time that adolescents develop new cognitive abilities, many middle schools ask students to do more ROTE tasks that are LESS cognitively demanding. Whereas elementary school projects often ask kids to integrate and think creatively about material, middle schools often ask kids to memorize and repeat back information. Although there are many good reasons for this - you can't think integratively and intelligently in the absence of facts and solid knowledge, it can also be frustring for students who feel that they are doing more repetitive, less challenging tasks. Math, in particular, tends to focus on review and consolidation rather than learning new skills.

Thinking about multiple possibilities can cause kids to freeze. Presented with many different possibilities, kids can freeze up, spending more time thinking and deciding than choosing a path and doing.

School's demands for organization may outstrip kids' abilities to do it. Moving from class to class requires kids to rapidly adjust to the expectations of different teachers. Assignments are rarely as integrated as they are in elmentary school or as teachers would like them to be. And the physical act of bringing home all those books and all those papers - and getting them back again - can be daunting.

The responsibility for completing their work lies in your child

It is important to remember that the primary responsibility for completing work well is with your child. But it's also really easy for us to believe that when they don't immediately do that well, it's from stubbornness, or laziness, or lack of effort.

Begin with the assumption that it's not. Most kids want to do well. They certainly don't want to get in trouble and don't want to spend more time on their homework than they have to. Giving them the tools they need can improve homework quality while at the same time reducing the time it takes to complete it.

Some strategies that work

Parents can help kids get organized by focusing on the PROCESS and LOGISTICS of school and not just 'helping with homework' and working on content. By focusing on HOW they do their homework (what time, what conditions) not the content of it, you let them keep control over it while giving them tools to manage it effectively themselves.

In addition to these suggestions, go to this page on Children With Special Needs for a wealth of additional information. A list of strategies for both teachers and parents are available here at Intervention Central.

Where things fall through the cracks.

When my son and I went through his problems with completing and turning in his work, we came up with five key points where things fell apart. These were the principles we arrived at:

- Eliminate thinking as much as possible
- Make organization automatic
- Use planners or assignment books effectively - you can't count on memory
- Make sure all materials are home when they're needed
- Make sure completed assignments can be found and TURNED IN

Make things automatic. The single most important thing you can do is to help your child make good organizational skills AUTOMATIC. The less they have to think, the less likely they are to make mistakes. The goal is for good organizational skills to become habitual so your child doesn't have to think about and remember what to do. They go to class, sit down, and open their planner and check the board for assignments.

Organize all materials together in one place. When my son got his supplies list at the beginning of the year, he was asked to get 7 folders and 7 spiral notebooks, plus two three ring binders. The idea, I know, was to minimize what the kids had to carry back and forth to school. Kids are supposed to bring home what they need and leave the rest at school. This only works for organized kids. For my son, it meant that he'd always be home without the notebook he needed to do his homework.

A few years ago we had solved the problem by putting everything into one humungous three ring binder.

Last year, that didn't work, as the folders and notebooks were just too numerous. After six month's experimentation, we finally got a new system: a large expanding accordian folder that took file folders and spiral notebooks alike. It even took his assignment book.

This year EVERYTHING went on an iPod Touch. He takes pictures of the assignments the teacher writes on the board. .He takes pictures of the worksheets so he can't lose them. He takes pictures of his assignments so he can print them out again if (when) he loses them. He enters his assignments in an app that is fantastic for keep track of assignments. He does his writing assignments on Google Docs, which are accessible from anyplace that has internet. He shares them with his teachers or can access them from his iPod and print them out. His teachers (bless them) will also let him just show them the picture and give him credit.

Which system works for your child may differ. But the idea is simple: if everything is in the same place and goes back and forth from home to school, materials are at home when needed and completed work goes back to school where it can be found. It's one less thing to remember. If you buy thinner notebooks and eliminate completed work, it isn't too much to carry.

Assignment books are the critical first step in making sure that homework is done. Many kids' metacognitive skills haven't caught up with the fact that the complexity of their tasks has outpaced their ability to keep everything in their heads.

WHAT THEY CAN DO:

Your child MUST keep an accurate list of assignments in their planner (paper or electronic). Many kids think they'll remember an assignment, because they haven't yet realized how hard it is to keep track of the many tasks they're assigned. Different schools use different methods. Make sure you understand the system that your child's school uses to record assignments so you can help them use it effectively:

- **The traditional method:** Write down the assignment on the day it is due. The way I and many parents were taught to use a planner is to write assignments down the day it is due. You look ahead and know what to work on. You can put in 'tickler' notes to break down long assignments into smaller parts.
- **A newer method:** Writing down an assignment the day it is

assigned. Both my sons - in two different school systems 10 years
apart - were taught to write down assignments on the day they are
ASSIGNED. After 10 years, I have finally learned how this
system is SUPPOSED to work, although neither of my sons ever
did. It does make sense and is an excellent system if your child
can use it.

- When an assignment is assigned, write it down the day
  assigned AND THE DAY DUE.
- The next day, check the previous day's assignments.
  Anything not complete gets written down again. Each day,
  continue to add new and uncompleted assignments. When
  an assignment is done, check it off.
- With this system, each day's listing works as a 'to do' list. It
  thus combines both an agenda and a to do list.

PHOTOGRAPH THE CHALK BOARD. Most of my son's teachers write
the assignments on the boards. Many of them have the week's assignments
written there on Monday. Take a picture. They can organize it later.
WHAT YOU CAN DO:

**Ask your child about each class and check to make sure any assignments
are written down.** Be especially aware of patterns. Is spelling always due
Thursdays? Math tests on Fridays? Put it on your own calendar so you can
remember to ask.
Check their planner against other sources of information. One way that
parents can help is to check assignment books against other sources
information to make sure they are complete. Your kids can do that too. Many
schools put some assignments on-line. Other teachers hand out calendars.
Others have weekly scheduled. For example, my son's Language Arts
teacher assigns spelling, analogies, and grammar on Monday, Tuesday, and
Wednesday, respectively, and everything goes in on Thursday. Writing that
down at the beginning of each week helps to keep things in order.

If it's still not working, ask for help from the school. If, after all best
effort, you child still isn't bringing home an accurate list of assignments,
enlist help. Ask your child to stop by their teachers after school or at the end
of each class and check their assignment books. If your child isn't turning in

homework, your child's teacher is probably at least as frustrated as you and your child.

Make sure needed materials are home when they're needed. One of the real challenges of getting homework done is making sure that each of the books, handouts, and assignment lists are home when they're needed.

WHAT THEY CAN DO:

Check the assignment book at the end of each day as they're packing for home.

Set up a system to remember books. Have your child mark down what they need when they write down the assignment. For example, they can put a post-it note on the front of the planner. When they write down the assignment, they write down the books or handouts they need to do it on the post-it. If they check their post-it before they leave at the end of the day, they should be set.

Ask for extra books. Is this a chronic problem? Does you child have a 504 or IEP or just concerned teachers? Ask for an extra set of books. In addition, many books are available electronically and the teacher just have to give you an access code.

Don't forget worksheets! Sometimes putting all worksheets directly in the planner is the best way for them to make it home. My son takes photographs of every worksheet he is given so it's on his iPod, he can't lose it, and he can print them out if they get lost.

WHAT YOU CAN DO:

Still not working?

If you can get a second copy of your child's books, DO IT. Some books are needed every day, but others are only needed once in a while. Kids often forget books not needed on a daily basis. This can cause major problems. It had never occurred to me that I could solve this problem by getting an extra copy of textbooks, but when I asked, my son's teachers were happy to oblige. Often now they are available electronically, you just need to get the passcode. If you're having a problem, they may have extra copies of old textbooks stuck in a closet somewhere. Ask. They can only say no.

Turning in Completed Homework

Maybe it's just my family, but both my sons and two of my nieces complete their homework and then never get credit for it because they (a) leave it in their locker (b) can't find it when they teacher asks for it or (c) forget to turn it in. Because teachers are trying to reward good homework skills, this often means 0's entered into their grades or, when we're lucky, losing half the credit or more. Frustrating.

WHAT THEY CAN DO:

Put all homework in their assignment book. For some children, slipping all homework for the day into their assignment book is a good strategy, as they need to take it out to write down their new work. If that works, go for it. Flag assignments that will be turned in.Because some homework needed to be in binders and other was loose, keeping it all in one place simply did not work for my son. Flags did. You know those bright post-it notes or flags you can buy? Or paper clips? Every time my son completes an assignment, he puts a bright flag on it before he sticks it in his accordian folder. When he opens the folder up, the first thing you see is four or five bright markers, showing what has to be turned in for the day. Since he began using this system, he hasn't lost one assignment.

Have them photograph every assignment. The ones they do in class. The ones they do at home. My kids can lose anything. Photograph it. They may also realize the assignment they thought was done wasn't finished. The photograph will show it to them.

Do all work that can be done in Google Docs. They can't lose an assignment typed into Google Docs. They also can't lose an assignment photographed or scanned and uploaded to Google Docs. Anything in Google Docs can be printed again. Many teachers who are just checking off that things are done will just look at an iPod or phone and check it off as there.

WHAT YOU CAN DO:

Essentially nothing. You can teach your child strategies and give them the tools they need to do their work. You can make sure they photograph or upload it. But ultimately, once the homework is done and they are off at school, they're on their own.

The Disorganized Child

The New York Times published a piece by noted psychologist, Alan Sroufe, about the long-term problems of relying on ritalin to help kids who have problems with hyperactivity and concentration in school. Bottom line: it doesn't work. Whatever your feelings about the diagnosis or over-diagnosis of attention deficit disorder, ALL of us need tools to help us stay organized and on-task in this very demanding and multi-tasking world.

Middle school is a great place to learn skills that can carry kids forward into adulthood. Some kids may develp those skills naturally. Other kids need some help. But all of us can benefit from making good strategies automatic, so can work more effectively.

Disability? In College? Advice on Talking to Professors

Explaining your disability can get you more effective help from professors[.]

The Americans With Disabilities Act (ADA) protects students with conditions that impede normal life functions from discrimination (The American Psychological Association's Summary can be found here). "Normal life functions" include going to school. I know much more than I want to about this act, because my son is chronically ill from one of many invisible illnesses. He has severe, chronic migraines that leave him in pain much of the time. The American with Disabilities Act also protects children with Attention Deficit Hyperactivity Disorder (ADHD), depression, and a host of learning disabilities. In elementary and high school, the accommodations needed to help people who face these barriers get a fair chance at education are covered by IEPs and 504 plans. These plans lay out what the student's, parent's, teacher's, and school's responsibilities are in creating a successful learning environment for the student.

When children are younger, this is usually managed by the parent. But as kids enter college, they take on the role of managing their own learning themselves. In fact, they have to—it is against the law for professors to talk to parents about their child's education without explicit permission from their student.

I've taught at seven colleges and universities over the last 30 years (I feel old now) and they all work about the same. I don't know how the process of getting an IEP and accommodations works specifically in different colleges. I do know what I get handed by my students. Some students do a superb job managing disabilities. Others not so much. There are many other resources available to you written by people who have disabilities or who have spent their job fighting for fair access. I am not an expert on disabilities—I'm just the mother of someone who suffers from one. These are just my thoughts as an professor on how students can really help me to help them get the education they deserve.

Don't just hand your professor your accommodation letter

When students register with the college or university office of disability services, they are usually evaluated and have their disability and needs documented. Then they are typically given an accommodation letter, saying what changes they may need from normal classroom procedures in order to succeed. For example, a typical student with ADHD will give me a letter saying they need time and a half for exams and that they need to be in a quiet room free of distractions.

LOTS of students (almost all of mine) just hand accommodation letters to me and leave. If I ask them what they need specifically, they kind of shrug and say 'taking the exam in a separate room—you're already doing everything else I want'.

That's not very helpful if they have a complicated disability like migraine or depression or many other invisible illnesses. To maintain privacy the accommodation letters are really general. They don't give a diagnosis. Sometimes they say generally the problems students have, but not in enough detail for me to know what to do. For example, they'll say 'problem processing abstract cognitive material'. This is a college. What does that mean in term of what I can do to help them learn what I'm teaching? The letters do say concrete things like "Time and half on exams. Quiet testing space without distractions." But that's not enough to help someone with diabetes, migraines or depression, for example, who is going to miss classes some days, who needs to eat in the middle of an exam, or who needs a dark room or can't look at a computer screen on random days.

What you can do to help your professor help you

Make sure your full needs are in your letter. Let me be upfront about this. Many students with serious disabilities don't have the time or energy to do anything more than get to classes and do their best to get their work done. All you can do is hand that letter to the professor. If that's true for you, make SURE that your accommodation letter communicates all your needs. Are there likely to be times when you will be unable to work for a few days at a time and you will need an extension equivalent to twice the time you're unable to work? Put it in the letter. Do you need food at regular intervals - even in the middle of an exam and sometimes on short notice? Put it in the letter. Are there times when you can't look at a screen so won't be able to attend a computer lab? Put it in the letter. Don't let that accommodation letter be a rubber stamp - make sure it is individualized to cover what you think your needs are going to be.

Visit your professor early in the semester. I would strongly, strongly strongly urge each student to go to their professors' office hours at the beginning of the semester and explain the issues, before any problems occur. I know this puts an additional burden on peole who are disabled. That's why I suggest doing it early on at a time of your choosing, not when you're in crisis. I also know that it can be hard to reveal a problem that is deeply personal—especially one that is stigmatized. However, I know from experience that many students can successfully talk about their needs and the kinds of problems their disability causes them without telling me specifically what is the underlying cause of their problems (e.g., depression or anxiety). Do not feel you need to reveal private information about yourself. Make sure the professor understands your accommodation letter. But if there are specific, reasonable things that can be done to help you succeed, ask for it. Often much more can be done than is asked for in your accommodation letter.

Educate your professor. The more you can tell your professor about your disability and how it affects your academic performance, the better. I'll take migraines as an example. Most professors will not know what serious chronic migraines are in any meaningful way (I didn't.) What they know may be wrong in all the really annoying ways that people can be ignorant about disabilities. Just because someone is a brilliant physicist or an excellent Shakespeare scholar doesn't mean they know anything about your situation.

Talking to the professor and handing them a summary of your issues is very helpful. This can be part of your accommodation letter. For example, I wrote a useful summary for my son's high school teachers. It informs them about migraines in general and him in particular. You can write one for yourself. Or there are lots of excellent summaries online - attach one. If you're meeting in person, this gives you the opportunity to discuss behavior that professors might see as 'slacking' or 'lack of interest' as just problems related to illness. Trust me—when kids don't turn in work or don't show up for class, the professor's first thought is that they don't care or are drinking, not that they are sick. Going to the professor right at the beginning of the semester demonstrates that you are being pro-active and are working to succeed despite your handicap and are taking responsibility. Then if things go south, the professor will be worried and not annoyed.

If you aren't able to meet with each professor individually (see Spoon theory below), write them a letter or an email. Have it included with your accommodation letter. But do it early, before barriers arise.

Tell them about the Spoon Theory. If you have an invisible illness, you probably know about Spoon Theory. Spoon theory is a metaphor used by Christine Miserandino to explain why it's so hard to have an invisible disability. It gets through that unbearably frustrating belief that if 'you just tried harder' or 'pushed through' you'd be able to function okay. It helps people who have never had a disability or a serious illness understand a little more about your life.

The basic idea is simple. You hand someone 12 spoons. That's their energy for the day and that's all they've got. They take a shower—that uses up a spoon. They get dressed—another spoon. They make breakfast and put away the dishes—two more. It's really clear that every small, tiny little thing that everyone else takes for granted is much harder for someone who has a disability that robs them of energy. Lupus. Chronic pain. Headache. Depression. Anxiety. Hand the essay to the professor with the description of your disability (if you choose to reveal it) and your needs. It may help them 'get it'.

Ask for what you need. Letters from the Office of Disability at the college or university are probably pretty general. If you think you'll be absent a lot and at random, let the professor know up front. Set up a system ahead of time for what will happen when those absences occur. Every professor I know is willing to send Powerpoints to students when they are sick if they're asked to do so. Put it in your letter. Many of us—especially at big schools—record all the lectures so students who miss them can watch them online. See what resources are available. They may already have everything you're going to need. Wouldn't that be a relief?

Students can also request from disability services someone who will record the lecture for them if they miss it. In many schools, students can be paid to record lectures or take notes if this is not already a normal part of college routine (in many large schools, it is). It might also be to the students' advantage to show the professor how to record lectures themselves. It's really easy. On a Mac you just use the pre-installed Quicktime and start the record function at the start of the lecture. Your voice and everything on the screen (Powerpoints) are recorded and saved. On Windows you just download a free Microsoft utility for doing the exact same thing. If you know how to do this, it can help you help the professor help a LOT of students. It's not just students with disabilities who are helped by these simple, easy accommodations. It's busy parents. It's people holding down a job and going to school. It's students who have English as a second language. Most acommodations help everyone—not just people with identified disabilities. It creates an even playing field.

Most professors aren't jerks (some are). But explaining your issues and possible problems early and openly evokes most professors' protective instincts. And it's a lot easier for professors to help in advance than having them get annoyed because you seem disengaged and then explain later that, "no, I'm just really sick."

Remind them. Even the best-intentioned professor may forget who you are or what your needs are. Most professors have hundreds of students each semester. When I taught at a big school, I had thousands every year. When an exam is coming up and you will need a quiet space or extra time, remind the professor ahead of time so they can make arrangements. Standard accommodations will normally be taken care of, but if your needs are unusual, make sure people are ready to meet them. If you need someone to read to you because you can't see well that day, tell them early enough that arrangements can be made. When you realize that you are in blinding pain that morning, or throwing up, or are recovering from a seizure, tell them that you have a problem, but also remind them why you need accommodations. That's what the letter is for.

Get help from the administration. Finally—if you are having a bad week (or two), you probably have a Class Dean or Dean of Students whose job it is to notify all your professors. This is the time to get someone to do the work for you - contact one person and let them contact all your professors. For example, I'll get sent a note from a dean saying so and so is ill and will need help catching up. This notifies professors that this is a serious problem, that the student is trying their best, and that the dean expects the professor to be accommodating. If you don't have a dean, you do have an advisor. There is also someone in the Office of Disability Services whose job it is to help you succeed. Getting support from outside helps even with professors who are not as responsive as they should be.

One more hassle of having a disability

Constantly having to educate others about your disability is one of the many hassles of having one. But you have a right to an education free of discrimination. You have a right to have barriers removed. Unless people know what you need, they cannot give it to you. Pulling together a packet of information that says what you need and helps people understand what they can do to help may require less effort long term than trying to fix something once things fall apart. And once you pull it together for one class, you can hand it to everyone.

Parenting A Child In Pain: Both the Same and Different

Although there are many things that only a parent whose child is in pain can understand, parenting a kid who is sick is also just that: parenting. These essays talk about parenting more generally, but are ones I thought were particularly relevant when dealing with a child in pain.

Authoritative vs. Authoritarian Parenting Style

There's a big difference between discipline and punishment[1]

In response to the indictment last week of NFL player Adrian Peterson for child abuse, essayist Michael Eric Dyson wrote a thoughtful piece about the roots of corporal punishment within the American Black community.

Among many insights is the following quote:

"The point of discipline is to transmit values to children. The purpose of punishment is to coerce compliance and secure control, and failing that, to inflict pain as a form of revenge . .."

Dyson discusses the etymology of the two words. 'Discipline' comes from the Latin "discipuli," from which we get the word 'disciple.' 'Punishment' comes from the Greek 'poine' and Latin 'poena,' which means revenge, from which we get the words 'pain' and 'penalty.'

'Discipline' I find to be an interesting word with regards to parenting. It connotes one who shares the beliefs of a master and who follows their teaching. It also connotes being able to stick to a difficult path, despite temptations, as in the phrase 'self-discipline'. The distinction between discipline and punishment come out clearly, I think, in how we use the two phrases 'self-discipline' and 'self-punishment'. The first is a strength. The latter dysfunctional.

Self-punishment and self-discipline mean very different things

Psychologists classically describe overall ways of parenting in terms of parenting styles. The most commonly used typology of normal parenting is based on work by Diana Baumrind. She distinguished between Authoritative, Authoritiarian, and Permissive parenting. (Later, Maccoby and Martin developed a typology of parenting based on Baumrind's work, and added a Neglect/Abuse category; parenting style typologies do not address abusive or pathological parenting).

Unlike later typologies of parenting that were melded onto her work, Baumrind focused on control: she believed the job of parents is to socialize and teach children. Parents differ, however, in the type of control they exert. I want to focus on Authoritarian and Authoritative parenting, as these two styles really differ along that idea of punishment v. discipline. (The other two types of parents - permissive and neglectful - are both relatively low in control and socialization attempts.)

Authoritarian parents believe that children are, by nature, strong-willed and self-indulgent. They value obedience to higher authority as a virtue unto itself. Authoritarian parents see their primary job to be bending the will of the child to that of authority - the parent, the church, the teacher. Willfulness is seen to be the root of unhappiness, bad behavior, and sin. Thus a loving parent is one who tries to break the will of the child.

Baumrind's exemplar of an authoritarian mother is Susanna Wesley, mother of the founders of the Methodist Church. She writes

As self-will is the root of all sin and misery, so whatsoever cherishes this in children ensures their after-wretchedness . . . whatever checks and mortifies it promotes their future happiness and piety.

Wesley's discipine was "strict, consistent, and loving," clearly motivated by her love for her children (Baumrind's original description of authoritarian parenting with supporting quotes can be found on page 891 here.).

Authoritative parents are also strict, consistent, and loving, but their values and beliefs about parenting and children are markedly different. Authoritative parents are issue-oriented and pragmatic, rather than motivated by an external, absolute standard. They tend to adjust their expectations to the needs of the child. They listen to children's arguments, although they may not change their minds. They persuade and explain, as well as punish. Most importantly, they try to balance the responsibility of the child to conform to the needs and demands of others with the rights of the child to be respected and have their own needs met (see page 891, above)[a].

My students have always had trouble with the words 'authoritative' and 'authoritarian' because, over the years, they have come to be used almost synonymously. But they are fundamentally different, just as the words 'punishment' and 'discipline' are. Authoritative parents teach and guide their children. Their goal is to socialize their children so they come to accept and value what the parents value. They hope their children will internalize their goals. They are shepherds. The word 'authorative' was chosen to imply that parents have power because they are wiser and are legitimate guides to the culture.

Authoritarian parents, however, exert control through power and coercion. They have power because they exert their will over their children.

Interestingly, authoritative parents tend to be MORE strict and MORE consistent than authoritarian parents. They set fewer rules, but are better at enforcing them. The children of authorative and authoritarian parents tend to be equally well-behaved and high achieving. The children of authoritarian parents, however, tend to be somewhat more depressed and have lower self-esteem than those of authoritative parents.

The language of parenting:
Legitimacy of parental authority

The words we use to describe parenting evoke strong emotions[.]

The language we use to talk about parenting tends to evoke strong responses both because parenting and our children are so important to us and because parenting so deeply reflects our values.

Although probably the first systematic study of parenting style was published by Symonds in 1939, research on parenting took on new urgency after World War II. How had so many people voluntarily participated in genocide? How had 'following orders' come to overrule all other human values? Where was the balance between raising a good, obedient child and one who could think for him or herself and act based on moral conviction?

In the years following the war, researchers identified three basic styles of 'normal' parenting: authoritarian, permissive (or indulgent), and democratic. Authoritarian parents valued obedience for the sake of obedience. Diana Baumrind, describing this style in the late 1960's, described authoritarian parents as believing that their job was to socialize children to act 'appropriately'. In other words, they believed a good parent was a parent who (lovingly) bent the child to their will. Objectively, authoritarian parents demanded compliance, but were relatively low in warmth. They set rules, but didn't explain them. Permissive parents, on the other hand, viewed themselves primarily as resources to their children. They saw their role as supporting the child and helping them to make good decisions. They provided guidance, but not guidelines or rules. Researchers characterized permissive parents as relatively high in warmth, but low in demandingness.

Interestingly, Baumrind changed the language psychologists had used to describe parents who were both warm and demanding from 'democratic' to authoritative. Authoritative parents set clear high standards for their children but were warm and supportive. They explained rules, listened to their children's arguments, and changed the rules when their kids made sense. When children acted responsibly, they were given more responsibility and greater latitude to make choices. In my favorite description of authoritative parenting, Baumrind describes it as helping the child to fit themselves to their environment so they can work and play well with others, while changing the environment to fit the needs and inclinations of the child. It should be noted that Baumrind basically argued that all parents wanted to influence and (dare I say it) exercise control over their children. They just approached it differently.

Baumrind and others have found that authoritative parents tended to be the warmest and most responsive of all parents, were the most consistent about following through with the rules they set (although they set slightly fewer than authoritarian), and had kids who tended to do well in school, keep out of trouble, and be both happier and more autonomous than their peers.

I love the word 'authoritative', although its meaning has mostly been lost to my students and it is difficult to translate into Chilean Spanish, where I do much of my research. My students think of the words 'authoritative' and 'authoritarian' as synonymous: harsh parents who unilaterally try to control their children through power assertion. But that isn't what 'authoritative' means. Baumrind chose the word well. Authoritative connotes legitimate authority based on knowledge and expertise. 'Authoritative' parents feel comfortable about settings rules because they know more than their children, have more knowledge of the world, and have the obligation to protect and nurture their kids. The children of authoritative parents tend to listen to their parents because they feel the parent is acting from their best interests and that they know what they're talking about. Authoritative parents get listened to, not because they are asserting power, but because their children have granted them authority and chosen to follow their guidance.

Which brings me to two key concepts: **legitimacy of parental authority** and **obligation to obey.**

Like the words 'authoritaritarian' and 'authoritative', the words 'authority' and 'obey' strongly connote unilateral power assertion. But, like many words in psychology, what the words could mean in day-to-day parlance isn't what they mean to psychologists.

Research on parental legitimacy and obligation to obey both grow out of really interesting work by Piaget on moral development. Piaget was one of the great psychologists of the 20th century. One of the many things that Piaget studied was how kids come to understand right and wrong. For example, young children base judgments of morality on how much damage is done, but older children judge moral harm based on intention. For a young child, accidentally breaking a tray of glasses is much worse than intentionally breaking one. An older child views an accident as fundamentally different from causing intentional harm – it is not a moral issue.

Similarly, young children see parents as having the right (legitimate authority) to control all aspects of their lives. Work by Turiel , Smetana, and others shows that kids say that parents can set rules over anything and that they are obliged to obey any rules parents set. These views change very quickly as kids enter elementary school. As they get older, children start to classify different issues as falling in different domains. For example, personal issues are those that affect only the actor. Moral issues are those that are right or wrong universally and based on an external system. Prudential issues are those that have to do with health and safety. Conventional issues are those that aren't moral, but rather have to do with following agreed upon social rules. Because of their social role as protector and caregiver, children tend to say that it is okay (i.e. legitimate) for parents to set rules about moral and conventional issues (hitting their siblings or swearing) and about prudential issues like wearing bicycle helmets. But kids are clear that parents have no right to set rules in the personal domain. Who their friends are, what kind of music they listen to, or what kinds of games they play are all off limits. Parents tend to agree: personal issues are off limits. What becomes complicated – especially as children become adolescents – is which issues are personal and which are conventional, prudential, or moral. Is cleaning your room a matter of personal discretion or a conventional (or, in extreme cases, prudential) issue? Is wearing jeans to church in the personal or conventional domain? Although who friends are and who adolescents date are prototypically personal issues, when does hanging out with kids who are clearly getting into trouble cross the line? One of my students suggested that for her parents, that line got drawn when, at 15, she started dating a 21 year old heroin addict. In retrospect, this seemed like a good decision to her. It didn't at the time.

Remarkably consistent cross-cultural research has found that, as children become adolescents and then adults, there is a normative expansion of which issues are judged to be in the personal domain. Prudential issues, such as judgments about what types of movies or tv to watch and judgments about health tend to get encorporated into the personal domain first. Drinking and substance use clearly move into that category. Interestingly, but perhaps not surprisingly, those are issues that youth typically say that their parents have the right (even the obligation) to set rules about, but that they are not obliged to obey.

Our own research suggests that although almost all kids show an age-related decline in the extent to which they believe parents have the right to set rules over different aspects of their lives, there are large differences between kids of the same age. We found that children whose parents were low in warmth, low in monitoring, and who are already engaged in some problem behavior at 12 had similar beliefs to kids with warm, high monitoring parents at 17. When we clustered kids based on their beliefs, we found that most adolescents did fall into the pattern Smetana had described: granting parents authority over prudential issues, somewhat over issues that combined the personal and prudential (hanging out with troublemaking kids), and not over personal issues like media choice, what they wear, or friends. But there were other kids who – even in late adolescence – believed that their parents have the right to set rules about all aspects of their lives and that they needed to obey the rules that parents set. And there are still other kids who believe parents don't have the right to set any rules. Interestingly, as we watch these children over time, most of them come to believe in the middle road: no to personal, yes to prudential. As adolescents become more cognitively sophisticated, as well as more autonomous, the distinction between what parents may do as part of their role as parents (e.g., tell their adolescents not to drink) and their own obligation to obey (I think I can drink responsibly) becomes sharper.

Smetana has shown that authoritative mothers draw much sharper distinctions than permissive or authoritarian parents between those areas that they set rules about and those they don't. More authoritative mothers tend to let their children govern their own personal lives and stay out of issues in that domain. Authoritarian mothers tend to define many issues others would define as conventional or personal as moral, and set rules about them. Permissive mothers tend define many issues that others would define as conventional or prudential as personal and thus set fewer rules.

Only setting rules about things that kids think are within parents' legitimate area of authority helps to add to parents' legitimacy and increase kids' feelings that they should obey the rules that are set. Legitimacy of parental authority and obligation to obey aren't things that parents assert. They describe kids' beliefs about those areas where parents are making rules because it's their job to and those areas where they should obey because it's probably a reasonable idea.

More reading . . .

- Baumrind, D. (1991). Effective parenting during the early adolescent transition. In P. A. Cowan & E. M. Hetherington (Eds.), Family transitions. Advances in family research series. (pp. 111-163). Hillsdale, NJ, USA: Lawrence Erlbaum Associates, Inc.
- Smetana, J. G., & Chuang, S. (2001). Middle-class African American parents' conceptions of parenting in early adolescence. Journal of Research on Adolescence, 11(2), 177-198.
- Nucci, L. P., Killen, M., & Smetana, J. G. (1996). Autonomy and the personal: Negotiation and social reciprocity in adult-child social exchanges. New Directions for Child Development, 73, 7-24.
- Turiel, E. (1983). The development of social knowledge: Morality and convention. Cambridge: Cambridge University Press.
- Darling, N., Cumsille, P., & Peña-Alampay, L. (2005). Rules, legitimacy of parental authority, and obligation to obey in Chile, the Philippines, and the United States. New Directions for Child and Adolescent Development, 108(Summer), 47-60.
- Darling, N., Cumsille, P., & Martinez, M. L. (2008). Individual differences in adolescents' beliefs about the legitimacy of parental authority and their own obligation to obey: A longitudinal investigation. Child Development, 79(4), 1103-1118.

Punishment is a powerful and effective parenting technique. But it works best when paired with rewards. It turns out that teenagers' brains, in particular, are much more attentive to rewards than to punishment. Using rewards can both be more effective and also make life a heck of a lot more pleasant.

Teens Respond to Pleasure, Not Pain: Parent Accordingly

Match your parenting to how teens' brains work[a].

It's not often that I read a scientific paper and immediately change how I parent my child.

But I did last week.

I was reading a series of pieces by developmental psychologist, Laurence Steinberg, first recipient of the Klaus Jacobs award for "groundbreaking contributions to the improvement of the living conditions of young people." Steinberg has spent his career studying adolescents. His early work focused on the family—how teens renegotiate family relations during the pubertal transition (kids win, moms lose) and then on parents' continuing role in adolescents' lives. His textbook, Adolescence, was the first in the field. It continues to educate generations of students who will go on to become healthcare workers, lawyers, and educators so that their work will be based on facts, not stereotypes.

More recently, Steinberg has focused his attention on adolecent risk-taking, integrating his training in human development and family studies with neuroscience and new brain imagining techniques. He was lead scientist of the amicus brief filed by the American Psychological Association in the U.S. Supreme Court case (Roper v. Simmons) that abolished the juvenile death penalty.

Last week, I read what Steinberg had to say about teenagers and risk.

Teenagers aren't stupid. Really.

Although teens are typically healthier than either children or adults, they wind up in the hospital a lot. Why? Risk. They crash cars because they're drunk or driving too fast. They shoot each other. They take foolish risks texting and riding bicycles. They get pregnant because they have unprotectect sex with condoms in their pockets.

Kids do dumb things. But they're not stupid. Study after study has shown that adolescents are AWARE of risks. If anything they are more aware of risk than adults are (probably because we keep warning them about danger) and overestimate the negative consequences of their actions.

Why then do they make foolish decisions?

It's all in their brains.

In Age Differences in Sensation Seeking and Impulsivity as Indexed by Behavior and Self-Report: Evidence for a Dual Systems Model, Steinberg and colleagues argue that the different growth speed of two areas of the brain create a perfect storm for risky behavior.

Their argument is straightforward. Sensation seeking—taking pleasure in strong positive experiences —is situated in two brain areas: the ventral striatum and the orbitofrontal cortex, both of which process incentives. Impulse control—what keeps us from acting prematurely—is situated in the lateral prefrontal cortex. Although both are involved in risk-taking, they aren't the same. Steinberg's analogy: people waiting in a long line at Disney World to take a roller coaster are high in sensation seeking (leading them to seek out risk) but also high in impulse control (which should help them avoid risk).

Although both areas of the brain change from childhood to adulthood, they don't change at the same speed.

The incentive processing centers become sensitized right after puberty, making adolescents take much more pleasure out of rewards. This leads them to experience risk as relatively more pleasurable.
The impulse control centers of the brain develop more slowly over time, and are still developing in early adulthood. This is the part of the brain that keeps you from doing risky things before you think through the consequences.
Too much accelerator, not enough brake

During most of the teen years, this creates a problem. Risky behaviors feel great and are experienced as more rewarding. Impulse control hasn't yet caught up—nor have knowledge and judgment. Thus emotion says go, but wisdom hasn't yet said stop.

How science changed my parenting

There are important take-home messages here for risktaking, social policy, and our understanding of teens that I will discuss in my next post.

But the first thing I took home from this reading had to do with my parenting. TEENS ARE MOTIVATED BY PLEASURE, NOT BY PAIN.

Thus telling a 13 year old that he will fail a test tomorrow if he doesn't study isn't that effective in inducing willing compliance. He knows that. But risk avoidance is not emotionally motivating. And that video game sure is.

Reminding a 13 year old how good it feels to accomplish something, how happy he'll be when he does well, and how much more time he will have to play if he studies efficiently works a lot better. Those POSITIVE emotions activate their incentive processing center. And teens are VERY sensitive to pleasure.

So I tried it.

I stopped reminding my son of all the negative consequences of not doing what he was supposed to.

I consistently pointed out how good it felt to do the right thing. Every positive I could think of.

A week later, things are going great.

He's less anxious. His work has improved. We've gotten along better. And he's taking more responsibility for making good choices. Even choices he doesn't like (like practicing his violin tonight because he wants a whole day of uninterrupted time on Saturday).

And you know what? I feel better too. I can be motivated by reward as well.

This is a touchy piece. It is based on several decades of outstanding work by Gerald Patterson and his colleagues at the Oregon Social Learning Center. It is about juvenile delinquency, but it is all too relevant to parenting a child in pain. Because just as we train them, they also train us. We try so hard to be supportive, that we can make it easier for them to do less than they can. Or the opposite happens. My son would struggle to make it into school and do a brilliant job of faking being well. And every time he did that, he got rewarded by being asked to do more work.

We can teach kids to show us their pain by only responding to their needs when they look helpless. And they can teach us to back off our demands by being so stubbornly difficult that it just doesn't seem worth it to ask them to try.

That's what this article is about. Trying to find a sweet spot between challenge and support. And remembering to both be fun to be around as well as that parent who pushes them out the door when they just want crawl under the covers.

How To Create a Juvenile Delinquent With Materials Easily Available At Home

Parents teach kids a lot - not all of it good[1]

The mom looked down, shocked, at her bare legs and worn underpants. She was standing at the edge of a crowded gym. Her 4 year old crowed triumphantly, holding the skirt he had just tugged to her ankles, his eyes on her face and ready to run.

She snatched up the skirt, snagged him by the waist, and strode from the room.

I never saw her again.

She had been asked by the YMCA instructor to watch her older son, who was maybe 8 years old. Her eldest was enrolled in a Tang Soo Do martial arts class. The teacher was having trouble with him, and had asked her to come to see if she could offer some insight and help before the son was asked to leave.

From the beginning, her four year old had been unhappy.

It was a big gym, with 20 or so kids lined up in disciplined rows from the most to the least experienced. The parents were huddled at the back, mostly sitting in the crowd of folded chairs, reading or talking quietly while they watched. Someone gave her a chair when she walked in, seeing how antsy her young one was.

He started out on her lap, but got up as she ignored his squirms. He played for a minute or so on the floor, then started wandering around and behind the gymnastic mats. After a few passes, he began to walk and then run faster and faster, back and forth along the end of the gym. His mom stood up next to the door, ignoring him, her eyes on the class. As he ran by, he would hit her leg and she would glance down, say hush, then turn her eyes back to her eldest.

Now his running was faster and more and more into the room. He started making loud swooshing sounds as he banked his turns. His hands become more grasping as he snatched at her skirt as he ran by.

She ignored him.

Finally, he ran up and stopped, grabbing the elastic waist of her skirt, and tugging it down. He looked at her expectantly.

The whole interaction had taken, maybe, 5 minutes.

It takes a lot of training for a child to be so effective at getting his mother's attention.

Gerri Patterson is a developmental psychologist who has studied parent-child relationships like this since at least the 1960's. His background is in traditional behaviorism and social learning theory, which he has used elegantly to help understand why sometimes parents can train their kids to act exactly how they don't want them to, and how some kids can train parents to parent them badly.

The tools are simply: reward, punishment, negative reinforcement, and modeling.

Psychologists use words very specifically and in ways that don't always match our day-to-day usage of them. To a behaviorist, the words reward, punishment, and negative reinforcement are defined by whether or not they increase or decrease the likelihood that the behavior that preceded them are going to happen again. It has nothing to do with whether reactions themselves are pleasant or unpleasant.

A **reward** is anything that increases the likelihood that a behavior will happen again. You give me flowers, I tell you I love you, you're more likely to give me flowers again. Saying "I love you" is a reward. Stealing a cookie and eating it without getting caught is inherently rewarding.

Punishment is anything that decreases the likelihood that a behavior will happen again. You give me flowers, I don't really pay attention, you're less likely to do it again. When my dog comes up to me expectantly, begging to go out, and I ignore her, it decreases the likelihood that she'll do it again (i.e., it is a punishment) and increases the likelihood that she will meet her needs in other ways (i.e., by peeing on the floor).

Negative reinforcement can also be thought of as escape conditioning. Here the word 'negative' means the absence of something (like 'negative space' in art – the space around an object). The key thing in negative reinforcement is that you are in a situation that you do not like. Getting away from that situation is rewarding. I yell at you. You leave the room and feel better. You hold a gun to me and ask for my wallet. I am terrified and hand it to you. You put the gun away. Your taking the gun away (withdrawing the aversive stimulus) is rewarding and makes it much more likely that the next time someone holds a gun to me I'll do whatever they say.

Negative reinforcement.

The tricky part of all this is figuring out which is which and in what situation. For example, if you study hard for a test and get a B, that grade is rewarding if you thought you were going to fail. It is punishment if you hoped for an A. If you had gotten drunk the night before and thought you were going to fail the test, not failing would increase the likelihood that you'd get drunk again before your next test.

Understanding what is a reward and what is a punishment is especially difficult when you're talking about something as complicated and nuanced as the interactions between kids and their parents. But it is really important to think about what is being taught (often accidentally and always by both parties) because parents and kids have hundreds of opportunities to reinforce each other's behavior every single day. Parents shape kids and kids shape parents.

By carefully following kids from toddlerhood into early adulthood, Patterson has found that the kids who grow up to get in trouble – arrests, drug use, and jail time – tend to have experienced a particular pattern of reinforcement. There are lots of other ways to grow up to get in trouble too, obviously, but this is one clear pathway.

It begins before the child even starts school.

Step 1: Begin with a lively, active, stubborn, or difficult child.

Step 2: Teach the child that disobedience makes rules go away.

It's easy. Ask them to put away their toys. When they don't, ignore it and pick them up yourself. Or yell at them, but don't make them do it. If they cry or whine or yell, tell them they can do it later. Or tomorrow. When they hit their brother instead of picking up the toys, send them both upstairs in separate rooms, where their other toys are. All parents do this sometimes. Parents whose kids grow up to get in trouble tend to do it a lot.

Step 3: Let the child teach you not to ask them to do anything they don't want to and not to correct them when you don't like how they behave. It is exhausting working with an uncooperative kid. Why ask them to turn off the tv, when last night it wound up in a two hour tantrum that left you both exhausted and angry? One of the most important steps to training a kid to behave badly is simply to stop trying to parent them because it is so, so hard and it never seems to work. Reinforcement works in both directions. And the more you've trained them not to listen, the better they can train you not to parent them.

Step 4: Fail to reward behaviors you like. Or, better still, punish good behaviors and reward bad ones. This is both subtle and important. When you've had a hard day and your child is playing happily – or even just zoning out in front of the tv – sometimes you just want to ignore them, hoping that it will last just five minutes longer.   Parents whose kids tend to get into trouble ignore their children when they are well behaved and only pay attention to them they are bad. Bottom line: if you want attention, you've got to misbehave. The cliché that you should try to catch your kids being good has a lot of truth to it.

Parents can take this a step further by inadvertently punishing their children for being good. The toddler brings you a flower and you dismiss it as a dandelion. They proudly show you their drawing and you criticize the way they drew the tree. They swear at you and you laugh at the incongruity or tickle them when they hit you.

Step 5: Let the child teach you that they're not fun to be around.

Having carefully failed to teach the child to behave appropriately and to become difficult and stubborn whenever things get hard, they're ready for school. This is a tough transition, because school is a place where kids spend a lot of time getting asked to do tough things that they don't want to or that are hard for them at first. So what happens next?

Step 6: The child misbehaves in school and doesn't learn well.

The child has learned that when they are asked to do something they don't like, they can ignore it and they won't have to do it. If that doesn't work, they can make a fuss and distract the adult so they can get some attention. Not good attention, but some is better than none. All of this takes away from the hard work of learning. And it does nothing for their relationship with the teacher either.

Step 7: Kids who behave well and do well in school won't play with the child.

In elementary school, most kids love their teachers and want to do well and be good. Kids who get in trouble are rejected by their peers.

Step 8: The child begins to hang out with other kids who get in trouble.

These new friends tease them when do what the teacher asks, don't respond positively when the child acts friendly, and laugh appreciatively and sympathetically when the child tells them about his escapades and misbehavior. And more learning occurs.

So now we have child who is in late elementary school or middle school, when lots of kids have new opportunities to get into more serious trouble that can get them in contact with the police or other authorities.

Step 9: The child becomes committed to his deviant friends, some of whom are older and already involved in more serious problem behavior, like drugs or drinking. Success at school or getting along with parents is not reinforced. The kids laugh uproariously at tales of misdeeds – real, planned, or imagined. They are scornful of suggestions that trouble be avoided.

And now you have a child with the real potential to get in serious trouble and without the skills they need to succeed in school or maybe even in the workforce. Their social skills – being pleasing, giving compliments, listening appreciatively and attentively – probably aren't well developed either, because those are not the social norms that help them with their group of friends.

Obviously there are lots and lots of places where this pattern can be broken. Some kids have easy temperaments and seem to move towards good behavior no matter what happens to them. Some kids are shy and, although they don't do well in school, also don't like hanging out with the rougher crowd of kids who tries to befriend them. Sometimes there are just no troublemakers for them to hang out with – and this might be the best thing that ever happens to them. Some kids wind up with great friends or talented teachers who bring out their best and teach some of the skills they were initially lacking. There are many turns off of this path. But lots of kids stay on that path all the way to the end.

You can see the patterning the Patterson described in the mom and her two young sons.

The mom brought her youngest into a situation where he was going to be bored without any plans for keeping him quiet or amused. (I think half of the problems that kids have come from putting them in situations where it's just plain hard for them to behave well.) When the child started to misbehave, the mom ignored him, so running around was more rewarding than not running around and had no negative consequences. The only time his mom noticed him at all was when he ran by and hit her (thus reinforcing the behavior). As his behavior got wilder, she ignored him more and more, so it took more and more extravagant behavior to get him noticed. Then the spark of genius – grabbing the skirt. Getting yelled at isn't fun (and I never did hear her yell), but hauling down the skirt certainly got her attention. And he was no longer hanging out, bored, in the gym. Negative reinforcement. Even if the consequences later weren't good, that little bit of learning was going to last.

Might another child with the same mom have laid down and fallen asleep or whined quietly or read a book or started up a game with one of the other waiting parents? Sure. But that's not this active child's temperament. It's not what he brought to the situation.

Interestingly, the reason the mom was there in the first place was because her older son was doing the same thing in class. Not pulling down the teacher's skirt, but acting aversively so that he didn't have to do what he didn't want to do, and getting a lot of attention by being bad.

This Tang Soo Do class, like every good martial arts class I have ever seen, was very disciplined and organized. Most young kids sign up for karate classes because they're all excited about flying kicks, punching each other, spinning leaps, and breaking boards. That's not the first thing they get. This class begin with bows, lots of pushups, and group recitation of shared values (seeing a group of teens and preteens shouting "Obedience to parents!" always cracked me up). Kicks and punches were carefully taught under very controlled conditions. Sparring was carefully monitored and no or low contact. Kids who were caught fighting outside of class were disciplined or asked to leave the program. Hard work and lots of encouragement and praise were the norm.

When the mom's 8 year old entered this class, he began cheerfully and enthusiastically, like the other kids. But when he got to his 10th or 12th pushup, he'd start to fade and then lie with his chest on the mat. The teacher would come over and encourage him. No, he couldn't do more. His hand hurt. The instructor would nod and tell him to join in on the situps. No, he was feeling a little sick. Jogging around the gym? "My leg hurts. Can I just sit out?" Now it's time for learning punches. After the exercise, the least experienced kids are paired with the older students so that things don't get out of control and are carefully monitored. "Oh, I didn't mean to hit you." "Did I just kick you in the stomach?" "Me? I wasn't laughing when that guy got hurt!"

The instructor for this class was really impressive in his ability to keep these kids happy and working hard. He gave kids responsibility and made every kid feel like they were doing their best, that their hard work was appreciated, and that he was proud of them. Now this one child was taking a quarter, maybe half of all his time and attention in each and every class. None of the experienced students would work with him because he didn't listen, wouldn't do what he was told, and kept hurting them and smirking that he was sorry. He couldn't work with the less experienced kids, because he distracted them and got them in trouble too. So his mom was asked to come in.

And that's where our story began.

And that's what Patterson sees when kids move from home to school and into the peer group.

Invading Privacy in the Name of Safety

Parents invade privacy too[1]

Privacy is big news. Or loss of privacy is.

We give away our privacy on Facebook. The Patriot Act allowed the US government to scoop up phone records en masse, a practice Congress now debates. And every time we give in to the convenience of swiping a card through a machine, we leave a trail of information that tells someone - businesses, schools, government - where we are and an enormous range of information about our interests.

Since at least the 1950's, public libraries have refused to release information about what titles patrons borrow, because it tells 'authorities' too much about our interests and private thoughts. Google has no such compunction.

Privacy and parenting

I was thinking about privacy this morning when chivying my son off to school. Chivying (a wonderful word - particularly applicable to the parents of migraineurs - that means repeatedly telling someone to do something) because once more my son had woken up in pain. The weather was beautiful but by 7AM we had already moved from fog to storm to beautifully clear. The barometric pressure had shifted with these fashions. And my son's brain - beautifully attuned to the nuanced shifts of our atmosphere - was wracked with pain: his skin hypersensitized to touch, his pupils wide open and way too vulnerable to light, cringing from sound, throwing heat, muscles tense.

Unlike short term illnesses, where rest is your body's best recourse, pain management centers around the country recommend people suffering from chronic pain and chronic sensitivities to go out into the world with their pain. Like Gollum in his cave, when people who are hypersensitive draw away from the pain of sound, sight, and touch, they become increasingly sensitive over time. He needed to get out into the world.

So once more, I was pushing my son to eat, get dressed, and get out.

Awkward for a mother of a teen boy. In fact, I shamelessly use that awkwardness to my advantage: I have handed him clothes and told him I'll put them on myself if he doesn't get himself dressed in three minutes. An effective threat I have never had to carry out.

My job as a parent is to ensure his safety and in parenting, safety trumps the child's right to privacy. But he has a right to privacy - certainly physical privacy in his person. Where is that line? At what point does concern for his physical health trump his right to privacy? Because he uses my unwillingness to cross lines of privacy to his advantage too. His war with pain is a battle where we are both allies, share common goals, but have different priorities in terms of long term strategies and short term tactics.

Legitimacy of parental authority

When parents and children talk about what areas it is 'okay' for parents to set rules about, what areas they 'should' set rules about, and which rules children 'must' obey, we are talking about an area of research on the legitimacy of parental authority. Growing out of Piagetian research on morality, it is about right and wrong. The job of parents is to protect and socialize their children. But that power is not unlimited.

Children, similarly, have a right to privacy and autonomy.

I have a right - a duty - to help my son restore his health and go to school. In fact, I have a legal obligation, placed on me by the state. But he has a right to make decisions about his person and to maintain his dignity and autonomy.

Over the past 60 years, we have learned that parents and children both agree that parents - incumbant on their role as protector and socializer - have the right and obligation to set rules and expectations about:

- **prudential** issues of health and safety (don't drink, look both ways before you cross the street, brush your teeth)
- **moral** issues (don't steal, bully, or hit your sister)
- **conventional** issues (no feet on the table, clean your room)

There are areas that empirical areas my colleagues find consistent support for that don't fall cleanly into those areas, but we call 'normal parenting':

- doing homework
- time spent on shared resources like common phones

There are areas that parents and their kids do NOT think parents should set rules about. These are defined as 'personal' issues and include areas that only concern the individual who is making the decision:

- choice of friends
- media use, like books, music, or movies
- hairstyle and clothing

But most areas of life fall in the cracks and are multi-dimensional. There are elements of multiple domains:

- That **homework** is done is something parents should ensure. How and when it is done is more personal (music on or off? on the floor or the kitchen table? immediately after school, before dinner, or before bedtime?)
- **Romantic relationships** are interesting because in all countries we have studied - the US, Chile, the Philippines, Italy, and Uganda - adolescents cede much more authority to parents about dating than they do in friendship. The personal is certainly there in terms of adolescents feeling they should have control of if and whom. But they also cede parents authority of some control over how and when - probably because issues of both covention and safety come into play. And those are areas of parental concern.
- **Problematic friends** are also an intersection. "Problematic" suggests prudential danger, but friends are clearly personal. Who gets to judge what is 'problematic'?
- And **media use** is also complex. Violence or pornography falls into the prudential or moral camp. But how much? What type? And does TIME spent on a computer when the child has already completed their other work constitute an infringement of the child's choice of leisure or a safety issue?
- **Alcohol and substance use** are always interesting issues, because they are almost unique in late adolescence because teens say that their parents should set rules about them - it's their job to tell them not to do drugs or drink. But they do not feel that they

should have to obey those rules. Most teens consider it an area of personal decision-making.

- **Sexual behavior** is also interesting, because they cede parents right to be concerned about their physical health and sometimes consider it to be a moral issue and thus of parental concern. But it is a deeply personal area that they do not concede decision-making power over.

Privacy and Parenting

Privacy and legitimacy of parental authority are deeply connected, because they are, at heart, about the integrity of the self. All people have an inherent right to dignity and control of their private thoughts and their sense of who they are. I believe this is at the core of the personal domain. No one has right to tell you what or who to like or how to spend your free time. That defines who you are. Reading a diary or email or scrolling through someone's photo scroll or texts is crossing a boundary from thoughts and decisions that concern no one but themselves into those they choose to share with others. I have written before about those boundaries and how they can be broken and shared in the post Sharing Privacy and Secrets Betrayed.

But sometimes the obligation to protect trumps the right to privacy. And that is the constant dilemma of parenting at the edge. A few years ago, a student of mine who was also a parent had a child who she thought was cutting herself. The child was 12. My student thought she was cutting her feet with a razor, although the child carefully covered her feet at all times and was loudly indignant at any suggestion that she was engaged in self-harm. My student eventually checked her feet and took her to get help when she found she was hurting herself.

Invasion of personal privacy? Prudential parenting? To me, the concern for protecting the daughter's health clearly trumped the daughter's right to privacy in an area where she was hurting herself.

But cases get fuzzier. Is parental concern that a child is engaged in sexual behavior one that warrants intervention? If the child is 10 certainly. If they are 16? If the issue is abuse or lack of contraception? If it is a moral concern? What about consensual sex in a romantic relationship?

The boundaries of child privacy and parental obligation to protect and socialize change not only over domains, but also with age. Research has clearly shown that both parents and adolescents cede more privacy to adolecents and less legitimacy to parents as children become adolescents and finally adults. But adolescents, at least, also differ. Some enter adolescence at age 12 essentially saying their parents have no right to set rules over anything - everything is personal and private. Others enter adolescence ceding parents control over everything - nothing is private. Most - around 55% - say it is a mixed bag. One of the results of cognitive development in adolescence seems to be that adolescents develop a more nuanced understanding of parental authority. As they get older, more and more adolescents move from the extremes into the more nuanced middle ground.

Going to School and Government Prying

Which gets me back to pushing my son out the door and government prying.

My son is 16 and at some point soon, will be making healthcare decisions on his own. In fact, since he is 4" taller than me and outweighs me by 20 pounds, the only reason I can get him out the door is that I can talk him into it. He knows that it's better for him to go to school. This IS a battle we're allies in. My persuasion, chivying, and threats help him to do what he knows he should do. And there are days when he just can't, puts his foot down, and there we are. He grants me legitimate authority to make health related decisions. And that is shown by the long lengths he will go to argue me into persuading me to change my mind - as when he did not want to go on a new medication and convinced me to reduce his medication level instead as a trial. He was right and it was a good decision. I know many parents whose kids take control of their privacy and decision-making in other ways: by lying. So they pretend to take pills and hide them. This is a problem with many older adults and psychiatric patients as well.

Privacy invasion by the government is also done by consent - and by similar means. When done legally, it involves them persuading us to trade privacy for safety. In other words, changing an area of lives from the 'personal' to the 'prudential' domain. And like parents, one role of the government can be thought to be protecting public safety. There is greater concensus that this is a legitimate use of authority with regards to threats from outside the country than from within. Thus threats from terrorists or communists tend to work more persuasively with the citizenry than internal threats.

Research on legitimate authority has found very similar thinking controls the use of power by governments as by parents.

Parenting A Child In Pain Has Changed Me

Pain, Ambiguous Loss, and Acceptance

Acceptance means holding both a painful now and a hopeful future in our minds[.]

Death can be a harsh shock, as someone is ripped from us and is no longer present in our lives. It has a finality to it - that's part of the shock and much of the pain. But it is real and concrete. Ambiguous loss is fundamentally different, in that it is a loss where we are simultaneously confronted with two simultaneous states that can't be resolved.

- A husband is kidnapped and we don't know if they're alive or dead;
- A mother has Alzheimer's dementia and looks so much like the person who loved and cared for us, but doesn't know our name;
- A child is swept away by a flood and they cannot find her body;

In these example of ambiguous loss, we must hold two ideas - living or dead - in our minds and hearts simultaneously. (See a discussion by Pauline Bloss on ambiguous loss and the myth of closure.)

Ambiguous loss can also be there when we hold two simultaneous ideas about someone we care about. A parent with dementia is an example of that - we hold in our mind both the person they were and the person they are. But we can have the same feelings about a child born with a severe disability. At every milestone, we may mourn the things they have not done - the first steps, graduations, and friendships that they miss - just as we celebrate and love the people they are and the accomplishments they have.

I was thinking about ambiguous loss with regards to the parents of children in pain. Because my own son has spent so much time in debilitating migraine pain, I have spent a great deal of time talking to other parents of children in pain. There are many wrenching emotions common to parents with severely ill children - guilt, anger, and helplessness loom prominent. But I also frequently hear just cries of loss for the life their child doesn't have - for the friendships not formed, the graduations missed, the proms left early, the sleepovers that never happened. And always this idea that their child has two lives - the one they are living and the one they would have had without the pain.

For kids in pain there are also two alternative futures - a future with the pain and one in which the pain is gone. Everyone's future can go in many possible paths. But this difference is particularly stark for kids who are chronically ill. Holding simultaneously to those two futures - one you need to plan for, one desired - is hard. Especially as a parent, where it is so easy to give in to guilt if that hoped for life without pain doesn't appear. There are so many imagined what ifs: What if I've chosen the wrong doctor? What if sending him to school is making him worse? What if there's a cure out there I've missed?

Acceptance

In pain circles, they talk a lot about acceptance. I have always thought of acceptance as learning to be comfortable with how things are. That's not something I am good at. Especially when what I thought I was supposed to get comfortable with is my child living in pain - forever.

I saw acceptance as passive.

In workshops this week for parents of kids in pain, though, I found I was wrong. They talked about acceptance as something active that one chose for the day.

TODAY I know my child is in pain. And today I will help him live the fullest life he can, taking that pain with him into the world instead of curling up with it in his bed.

In other words, learning to accept that the pain, right now, is their reality. Living with that reality - fighting to make their experience joyful in this moment right now - is acceptance. Knowing that tomorrow might be different. FIGHTING for tomorrow to be different. But putting most of one's effort into improving the NOW and living the NOW instead of waiting for something better in an ambiguous future.

That was a new concept to me. Thought of in this way, acceptance is an active verb, not a passive state.

Acceptance and ambiguous loss

Which brings me back to ambiguous loss. The defining quality of ambiguous loss is its dialectical nature. As with Schroedinger's cat, we must live with two antithetical potential realities. Living with a chronically ill child is like that. We have the reality of our child and the person they are and the life they live. They have been fundamentally shaped by their experiences and their illness is part of what has made them who they are. But we may also live with the life they might have lived without their illness - their ghost past. That is the child we may mourn.

Similarly, we fight hard for two possible futures: with and without pain. So I fight every day for my son to seize his day and put his mind and his self somewhere other than where his pain lives. THAT is acceptance. But I also hold part of my energy - my hope - into looking for another future reality for him: a future without pain.

Living in that dialectical future is hard. It takes a lot of energy. But doing so allows me to hold on to hope without sacrificing today for a maybe tomorrow.

What Not To Say to a Parent With A Child in Pain

Platitudes can hurt people in pain just as much as illness can

Emily McDowell has a series of empathy cards for people who have serious illnesses.

One of my favorites reads:

> *Please let me be the first person to punch the next person who says that everything happens for a reason.*

I can relate to that. My son lives in serious chronic pain from migraines and related headache disorder. He goes to school in pain. He eats in pain. He laughs and plays video games in pain. He has an amazing attitude and has gotten invaluable help and training from a clinical psychologist who specializes in working with children in pain. If you are in pain, I strongly urge you to find a good therapist who can help you to cope.

He has learned a lot from his experience. Yesterday, he told me he remains cheerful despite everything because he consciously focuses on aspects of his daily life that give him joy. That's where he keeps his self. In other words, he practices mindfulness as a conscious coping mechanism. As he heals—and I remain optimistic that he will get better—the skills he has learned will put in in good stead. If he can ever get his wheels off this sand, he will take off like a shot. This long miserable illness has helped to shape him into the amazing young man he is becoming.

But don't tell me that the constant agonizing pain he is in happened "for a reason." Or that maybe it's "for the best."

Keeping a Positive Attitude vs. Fatalism

Keeping a positive attitude and remaining optimistic is a critical part of healing for people who are chronically ill. For people in pain, in particular, depression at the limits it puts on your life is common. Depression causes pain, but pain also causes depression. The serotonin and dopamine levels and balance that contribute to one also contribute to the other. Pain can also lead to anxiety, as you constantly worry about how it will interfere with normal life functions.

Thus, maintaining a positive hopeful attitude, maintaining social relationships, and finding things that make you happy are important.

When my husband recently challenged someone who said that our son's pain happened "for a reason," she told him that he had to keep a positive attitude. But I don't think that believing his pain is part of a plan—of God, as this person believes, or of fate—is positive. It is fatalistic. It means that it has appeared for a reason and it will go away for a reason, and there is little that can be done about it.

It makes the person in pain a victim who can only suffer, like Job, who could do nothing to escape his fate.

To me, that is completely different than having a positive attitude. People with efficacy have a positive attitude. Warthogs—people who dig in and keep on pushing when the going gets tough—have a positive attitude. Similarly, people who believe that abilities are malleable and that hard work can increase intelligence work hard in the face of obstacles. They are positive and fight to hold onto their lives and keep going in spite of obstacles.

Efficacy is critically important for people to take action to maintain their health. According to Bandura's theory of social action, knowing how to do something is only one component of taking action to make your life better. You also need to believe that what you do will make a difference. Having a positive attitude enhances your belief that what you do makes a difference. Fatalism undermines it. It implies that what will be, will be, no matter what you do.

My son has a positive attitude. It helps him go to school in pain because he believes his doctors when they tell him it will help him recover. It gets him to exercise, drink lots of water, eat regularly, and stick to a very strict diet because he can see it help. IIe thinks his life will get better and that his actions and attitude will help him get there. That's a positive attitude.

I have seen what happens when kids lose that attitude in the sorrowful posts of mothers with kids very much like my son who are depressed and suicidal. If you've been in pain for years and you don't have hope, it must be hard to go forward.

To me, saying that illness and pain happens for a reason or for the best or that "there's a plan" takes away that efficacy. It tells me that there's a divine plan for my son to suffer. And I cannot accept that.

Section IV
Basics

If you're reading these essays, you probably know this. But a few more basics on migraine and pain.

Withdrawn, Irritable Teen? Is It A Migraine?

Pubertal migraines can look like nausea, irritability, or ADD

I've heard of migraines my whole life, but always as a kind of running joke featuring a stereotypical middle aged housewife. Then my son got them and I realized how devastating they can be. And that I had suffered from them as a teen as well

Migraines often begin and are most intense at puberty. They disguise themselves as many different illnesses, making them hard to diagnose, and even more difficult to treat.

They are brought on by common conditions that are experienced by many teens - hormone changes, stress, loud sounds, and lack of sleep.

Many people suffer migraines without headaches, and some of the symptoms look like our stereotype of teenagers: irritability, depressed mood, the desire to hang out in a quiet bedroom and just be left alone, being scatterbrained and having a hard time getting homework done, and just wanting to sleep.

Signs and symptoms

The classic migraine is an intense, throbbing, pulsing headache localized on one part of the head - often the temple. But migraines are much broader than that. Symptoms include:

- Headaches
- Nausea and vomiting
- Auras: floating spots of dots of lights or glowing auras around bright lights. Some people lose all or part of their vision.
- Painful sensitivity to sound, light and touch that makes being around people unbearable.
- A feeling of disorientation, lack of concentration, and 'spaciness'.

- Some people feel tingling, numbness, muscle weakness or are unable to speak clearly
- Some people tend to exercise particularly poor judgment just before or after a migraine.
- Severe migraines can be associated with hallucinations.

10% of people worldwide have migraines. They are three times more likely to strike females than males. They tend to spike at times of hormonal changes - puberty in both sexes and menopause in women.

Migraines usually last at least 3-4 hours and can last weeks. Most people with migraines have relatives with migraines or other related disorders.

Four phases of migraines:

The migraine cycle usually lasts for several days. It encompasses four phases: prodrome, aura, attack, and postdrome. The single most important thing to know about migraines is that the earlier you recognize them and take steps to prevent them, the better.

Prodrome:

Many migraine sufferers can tell a migraine is coming on a few days ahead of time. They experience:

- uncontrolled yawning
- depression
- food cravings
- hyperactivity
- irritability
- stiff neck
- constipation

Often, prevention at this phase can stop a migraine from developing. Most critical is quiet, low light, and sleep.

Aura:

Just before a migraine sets in, approximately one in three people experience auras. In additional to visual auras, these can also include feeling pins and needles, vision loss (often a blotting of the center of vision) or aphasia (difficulty with speech). Again, withdrawing from triggers at this phase (retreating to a quiet, dark room) can be critical in avoiding onset of a full attack.

Attack:

Migraine onset is often marked by nausea, loss of balance, extreme sensitivty to light or sound, as well as with a sharp throbbing headache. People often feel dizzy and experience blurred vision. They can be snappish because the world seems an overwhelming buzz of sensation (think drunk and dizzy at a midnight carnival midway).   Quiet and dark help.

The first 20 minutes appear to be critical. If a doctor has prescribed medication TAKE IT NOW. Once the migraine is established, it sets up a reinforcing cycle of pain that is difficult to break. Pain begets pain.

Postdrome:

After the attack, most people feel wiped out and spacey. Some people suffer from poor judgment during this period. Others experience mild euphoria.

Causes:

Like most headaches, the causes of migraines are poorly understood. They may be associated with changes in the brainstem interacting with the trigeminal nerve, a major pain pathway. They seem to be associated with serotonin imbalances - levels that are either too high or too low. According to the Mayo Clinic, the drop in serotonin levels during migraine attacks can trigger the release of neuropeptides which can irritate your meninges and lead to headache pain. Ironically, one of the drugs often prescribed to temper the vomiting of severe migraines is a serotonin suppressor.

Migraines can be triggered by growth spurts, by stress, lack of sleep, loud sounds and bright lights, physical activity, and changes in weather. They can also be triggered by foods, including nitrates and tyrmaine found in hot dogs and pepperoni, food additives common in snack foods, and cheese. A pepperoni pizza can be a migraine sufferer's worst nightmare.

Migraines at Puberty

A lot of migraine factors - especially changes in hormones, stress, and lack of sleep - are common characteristics of adolescence. We have just arrived at headache central.

One thing that makes migraines so sneaky is that often look like something else. Migraines often begin with feeling spacey, absentminded, and disassociated. Because migraine sufferers tend to be intensely sensitive to stimuli, they can be very irritable. They isolate themselves in their rooms to stay away from bright lights and sounds. This can be a good thing, because it can prevent the onset of a full bore attack. But it can also mask the fact that the problem is physical - a migraine - and not just a stereotypical teenage funk.

A migraine can also manifest itself as nausea. People with a migraine coming on can often feel a little - or a lot - sick to their stomachs. They may have little energy and be unable to concentrate. Younger adolescents will often experience migraine nausea without ever getting a headache, never realizing the underlying cause. Because nausea can be fairly regular - and migraines tend to be most intense in September (the beginning of school) and March (spring fever), it can look like a kid just trying to play hookey. They can't possibly feel sick to their stomach that often, right? This can seem especially suspicious to parents because migraines are often associated with tiredness and being unable to concentrate, so homework goes slow or doesn't get done.

For many girls, migraines come and go with their menstrual cycle, and are dismissed.

See a doctor - and things you can do for yourself

The NIH suggests that every migraine makes it more likely to have another migraine, so prevention is key. See a doctor early to get good advice on pain medication. Teens should also:

- Keep a migraine diary. Keeping a diary of activities that may trigger migraines can be the very best thing to avoid future attacks. It is also useful to bring to a doctor to discuss.
- Maintain a regular sleep schedule.
- Recognize the signs of an oncoming atttack. Often withdrawal to

a quiet place for even 20 minutes can stave off a full bore attack. Schools will often accommodate the need to leave class and lie down - there is often a sympathetic migraine sufferer in the main office. A doctor's note will help.

- Learn relaxation techniques. Relaxing jaws and shoulders can help relieve some of the stress that feeds into the nerves that trigger pain. Massaging temples and the joint joining jaw to skull also triggers pain relief in many migraine sufferers. And pain hurts less when you are relaxed.
- Think good thoughts. Surprisingly, research suggests that projecting strong positive emotions can also relieve migraine symptoms.

Chronic vs. Acute Pain

Most pain is useful. Chronic pain isn't[·]

When Benjamin Franklin wrote, "That which hurts, also instructs," he must have been thinking about acute pain. Because chronic pain doesn't instruct. It just HURTS.

Healthy, normal pain is part of all of our experience. It alerts us to injury. Without pain, we don't pull our hand back from a flame or realize our joints are twisted in ways that will dislocate them. Pain teaches us to avoid injury and tells us that we are injured and need to care for ourselves. The injuries and bodily damage experienced by people with leprosy are not inherent to the disease. Instead, they are caused when the bacteria that causes leprosy (Hansen's disease), destroys the nerve endings and thus the people's ability to feel pain. Children with familial dysautonomia cannot feel pain the way other people do, and it puts them in constant danger. Here is a description of a child talking about what it feels like when you feel no pain.

Acute pain alerts us to injury. But sometimes pain can take on a life of it's own. Chronic pain, on the other hand, may or may not alert us to an underlying tissue injury. For example, chronic back pain may be a sign of ongoing inflammation or injury. The pain from figromyalgia, on the other hand, is the result of the nervous system registering pain when no injury has occurred. It is dysfunctional pain, in that the pain is not alerting us to injury or disease, it is the disease itself.

One of the problems with chronic pain is that the nervous system becomes hyper sensitized to stimuli. Having felt pain, it is more likely to respond to other stimuli as being painful. Thus pain feeds on pain. For example, when my son is experiencing a severe migraine, all sensation is experienced intensely and as pain: wind on his cheek, the sound of a cat walking across the floor, light from weak sunlight on the floor. When chronic pain is left untreated, it can take on a life of its own and become more difficult to treat in the future. After an injury, for example, the area of the brain that interprets the pain can become hyperstimulated and continue to fire after the injury that originally started the pain is long gone.

The Pain Is In the Brain

Phantom limb pain is an extreme example of this. It is not at all uncommon for people to continue to feel a limb long after it has been amputated. In the absence of stimuli, the nerves that would normally interpret sensation from the limb begin to fire on their own, causing sometimes unbearable sensations of itching, burning, or pain. One of the more effective ways of treating such pain is to retrain the brain using mirror therapy. In this fascinating treatment technique, mirrors are arranged so that people 'see' their missing limb. Through careful manipulation, their brains are retrained so their sense of their limb is changed, causing marked reduction in painful sensation. The visual cortex seems key in mediating this treatment, drawing attention to the fact that pain is mediated through the brain, and does not reside in the injury per se.

Unfortunately, there are few effective techniques that work consistently for other forms of chronic pain. And chronic pain is common - even for children. Although older stereotypes say that infants or young children don't experience pain the way adults do, we know now that this is simply not true. According to Conquering Your Child's Chronic Pain by Lonnie Zeltzner, former director of the Pediatric Pain Program at Mattel Children's Hospital at UCLA:

- 20% of children 5-17 suffer from chronic headaches (15 or more headache days per month)
- 20% suffer from stomach pain 3 or more days a week for 3 or more months
- Juvenile arthritis, the most common chronic juvenile disease, affects 200,000-300,000 children in the US
- 6% of children may experience fibromyalgia, a condition characterized by chronic pain and fatigue, as well as mood changes.
- Chronic pain also accompanies cancer, a disease experienced by all too many children.

Children's pain not only causes them immediate suffering, but has important developmental consequences. It interferes with their ability to attend school, play, and engage in normal peer relations. We all know how hard it is to think when you are aching from the flu, have a splitting headache, or have sprained an ankle. Children with a condition associated with pain—migraines for instance—have a difficult time concentrating in school or engaging in normal cognitive functioning. In addition, many children and adolescents with severe chronic pain miss significant amounts of school. This takes a toll not only on them, but on their families as well. I have written previously about the experience of children who go to school in pain. There is the emotionally wrenching aspect of watching someone you love suffer when you can do nothing to help. But children's pain also interferes with caregivers' ability to work, can undermine sibling relationships, and can cause stress and discord between parents.

Pain kills. It is associated with depression, anxiety, and suicide.